THE
MILITARY MANUAL TO
STOP SMOKING ASAP
-
YOUR #1 MISSION

ACCEPT. ADAPT. ACHIEVE. ®

THE
MILITARY MANUAL TO
STOP SMOKING ASAP
-
YOUR #1 MISSION

ACCEPT. ADAPT. ACHIEVE. ®

JOHN H. CLARK III

BFG PRESS
HONOLULU

THE
MILITARY MANUAL TO STOP SMOKING ASAP
-
YOUR #1 MISSION

All Rights Reserved © 2023 by John H. Clark, III

Edited by
BFG Press
Published by
BFG Press
/ P.O. Box 2269 / Ewa Beach, Hawaii / 96706 /

www.BFGPRESS.com
ISBN 978-0-9820307-5-2

Printed in the United States of America

Accept. Adapt. Achieve. ®
is a registered trademark of John H. Clark III
All rights reserved.

COVER DESIGNED USING ASSETS FROM FREEPIK.COM

Success will depend on your commitment to the program, individual willpower, and other factors. This remedy might not work for everyone.

Medical disclaimer: Information presented in this book is not presented with the intention of diagnosing any disease or condition or prescribing any medical treatment. Information presented in this book is offered for informational purposes only. No responsibility is assumed by the author, publisher, or distributors of this information should the information be used in place of a licensed medical practitioner's advice and/or services. No guarantees of any kind are made for the performance or effectiveness of the preparations mentioned herein.

This book is available in quantity for promotions and charitable use. Send inquiries to info@bfgpress.com. (1) Portions adopted from *God's Heartbeat* © 2008; permission courtesy BFG Press. (2) Definitions adopted from wikipedia.com. (3) Statistics and facts from Center for Disease Control and Prevention - www.CDC.gov. (4) This book is not endorsed or supported by the Dept of Defense, the Dept of the Navy, or any other military or governmental agency. Information in this book is not official and has been voluntarily provided or is publicly available. (5) Brand names *Rio, Dorado, American Spirit, Marlboro, Newport,* and *Camel* are registered trademarks of their respective owners.

Regardless of whether your beliefs are right, wrong, or indifferent...

What you believe is true (to you)

John Clark III
Commander
United States Navy, Retired

☆ ☆ ☆ ☆ ☆

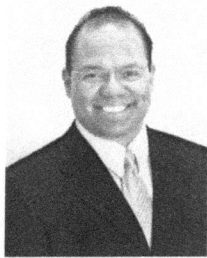

John H. Clark III
Commander
United States Navy, Retired

☆ ☆ ☆ ☆ ☆

I joined the Navy as a Data Systems Technician when I was 17, served for 32 years, and retired in 2018. I smoked cigarettes for over 15 years.

"The Military Manual to Stop Smoking ASAP" is a truth-based path to mission success in your effort to stop smoking. The methods within this book have worked for people all over the world. Using these methods, they all stopped smoking!

Today, this simple and effective method is yours. And, as you start your smoking-cessation plan, you should know the information herein should not be considered medical advice and is not intended to replace consultation with a qualified medical professional. I am not qualified to offer medical advice, and this book is not medical advice. Where medically oriented issues may be raised in this publication, I have offered my own opinion, and I do not claim professional or medical certitude, rigor, or competency.

Remember: any plan to stop smoking, including this book, must be evaluated in the light of your personal medical history and status. We recommend consulting a health professional about any proposed major change in lifestyle — including your goal to say, ***"I Quit Smoking!"***

THE MILITARY MANUAL TO STOP SMOKING ASAP

Table of Contents

"THE MILITARY MANUAL TO STOP SMOKING ASAP" is a short and very powerful manual. The last chapter of this manual is the next chapter of your smoke-free life. As the creator of your life, you write the next line; you draft the next chapter; and you are the hero of your own amazing story of success.

As you start a whole new life today, consider the awesome power you have within to change your world. Give yourself a new life! Take the next step, and write the final chapter of this book and the next chapter of your life in a true story that proudly says...
"I Quit Smoking!"

THE MILITARY MANUAL TO STOP SMOKING ASAP

Accept. Adapt. Achieve! ®

> *"Over the course of 15 years, I smoked over a pack a day.*
>
> *I **liked** to smoke; it relaxed me... or so I **thought**."*

After many, many attempts to stop smoking, I succeeded on December 31, 1999. I quit cold turkey and never picked up another cigarette. **You can quit smoking today** if you do three very specific things:

1. <u>Accept</u> a few facts.
2. <u>Adapt</u> your life to those facts.
3. <u>Achieve</u> what you want.

*Though seemingly simple, the methods offered in this small, but powerful book are directly responsible for helping people across the world immediately stop smoking. Thus, in my opinion, this single book provides all the steps **you** need to successfully stop smoking – **now**.*

Please note how short this book is. **This book is less than 50 pages**. That's very short! Reading this, you might wonder why I am highlighting the length of this book. To be honest, I am simply encouraging you to finish this book from beginning to end... straight through, in one sitting. If you truly want to stop smoking, make a choice to invest 45 minutes reading this short, powerful book - ***now***.

THE MILITARY MANUAL TO STOP SMOKING ASAP

As you read the following pages, notice the three words at the bottom of each page.

Accept. Adapt. Achieve! ®

To do anything and everything in life, we must accept a few basic facts about life. Sometimes those facts are known, but not yet seen. Sometimes, we must invest a little bit of faith in our acceptance of facts. Actually, faith is simply "accepting things not yet seen."

Will the sun rise tomorrow? We don't actually *know*, but we'd like to *believe* the sun will rise tomorrow. Our belief in the yet-to-rise sun of tomorrow is really an act of faith.

Will the U.S. dollar buy goods and services next week? We don't actually *know* this, yet we *believe* the dollar will sustain most, if not all of its value, over the next several years. Will a meteorite crash into my bedroom overnight? I don't know if this will happen… but I'd like to *believe* the sun will rise tomorrow; my money will still be worth what I think; and I will still be alive to spend it tomorrow.

Yes… EVERY thing requires a little bit of faith.

Yet, on the other hand, we walk a very fine line of daily denial, literally focusing on the day-to-day desires of today.

THE MILITARY MANUAL
TO STOP SMOKING ASAP

We pay more attention to our beliefs than to our knowledge. For example, there are more car crashes than air crashes every year. Yet, thousands of people are terrified to fly in an airplane. Exactly *why* are people afraid to fly?

Interestingly, instead of focusing on the **likelihood** of being in an accident, people tend to focus on the **survivability** of an accident. And considering the altitude of airplanes, if you ever are in an airplane crash, you will most likely perish in that airplane crash.

In daily life, however... given the sheer frequency and number of times you are in a car, you are much more **likely** to be in an automobile accident than an airplane crash.

Yet, most people who are afraid of flying are content to risk their life every day in a car. In reality, we are all in a soft sort of denial. We don't want to think about death; so we don't. We don't really care about *how* we will die... we simply know that we don't *want* to die.

Still, people who smoke are content to risk their lives every day in a fantastic dance with denial, believing something they know is simply not true. Do you *believe* or *know* your name? You *know* it, right? Know this: **smoking causes lung cancer. This is a fact.**

THE MILITARY MANUAL
TO STOP SMOKING ASAP

If...

If **you** are seriously interested in saying "goodbye" to cigarettes today, **you** must totally commit to changing your current thought processes. This is actually an easy and good thing to do. When **you** stop smoking, your life will change forever.

A few years ago, I was presented with information that has forever changed my life. I received a telephone call from my boss, and he told me my name was on a short list of potential *volunteers* to go to Iraq. I asked him when I was likely to fly to Iraq. His response shocked me. He simply said...

"They need you there next week."

One month later, I reported to the war-torn city of Taji in central Iraq, just north of Baghdad. There I was, in the blistering sands of time, facing a short-notice order to risk my life for someone else's principles, someone else's freedom, and someone else's life.

And when faced with such a vivid portrayal of The Valley of the Shadow of Death, I soon discovered how slight and razor-thin the edge of life actually is. I began to truly understand that life is but a heartbeat away from death.

THE MILITARY MANUAL TO STOP SMOKING ASAP

As you read the words on this page, death is but a heartbeat away. Do you care about your heart? Do you care about the life within you?

While in Iraq, I learned that my heart beats not because of any iota of my own doing. My heart beats not because *I* want it to beat. My heart beats because of the miraculous gift of life. Believe it; we are all living miracles.

And, as receivers of the tremendous gift of life, it is our responsibility to actively protect this great gift of life. Our fundamental mission is to present a style of life (a lifestyle) that will protect our bodies, prepare our children, and prolong our time with both.

Smoking cigarettes destroys your body and ultimately shortens your already limited time with precious people you love here on earth. That's a fact. As a smoker, you are risking your life for someone else's poison, someone else's profit, and someone else's principles.

Cigarette companies don't care about you, your life, or the fact that your money and your unhealthy lifestyle makes them filthy rich. The question is: **"Why don't you care?"**

"Quit Smoking Today!" can show you how to stop smoking if you want to stop – now.

THE MILITARY MANUAL
TO STOP SMOKING ASAP

War and Peace

"War is Hell."
~ William T. Sherman

I began my war training at the Army's Fort Bliss Post, in El Paso, Texas, on July 18, 2004. The temperature on my car thermometer reflected 100° F, a perfect location to gear up for the harsh extremes of the Iraqi desert.

Over the next few days, I was issued everything from a shovel to a pup tent, as I was equipped for hell on earth... a place for which there is no adequate preparation.

In the months before arriving in Baghdad, I had seen many presentations on the war in Iraq. And, given all that great information and intel, I actually thought I was well-prepared for war.

I had spoken to people who had returned safely from the war-torn country, and I really believed I had a "pretty good handle" on what I should expect in Iraq.

However, looking back, nothing (and I mean **not one thing**) could prepare me for ground-shaking mortars exploding everywhere around me... all hours of the day and night.

THE MILITARY MANUAL TO STOP SMOKING ASAP

Even the mass-marketed stories of combat displayed in the media could not delve into the smallest details of what it was like to be in central Iraq, in the thick of the battlegrounds. When I was in Iraq, the mortars fell in and around the forward operating base with a frequency far more than the frequency believed by the media and most Americans.

Remember: war is not a 9-to-5 occupation. And the enemy had no set time of attack. Mortars sporadically exploded in and around Taji at 2pm, 2am, and at almost every hour in between. Sometimes the small bombs exploded one at a time. During other attacks, the mortars fell one after another for as long as an hour or so... often longer.

After the bombings, there was a blackout period when all unofficial communication mediums were shut down, pending notification of next-of-kin for Soldiers, Sailors, Airmen, or Marines killed in the attacks. Telephone calls, e-mail, and all other unofficial communications were resumed only after family members had been notified.

On some blazingly hot, bright, and sunny days, despite the barrage of bombs, there would be no injuries, no deaths, and no shutdown in communications.

Those were the good days.

THE MILITARY MANUAL
TO STOP SMOKING ASAP

On most attack-filled days, though, there was an eventual quiet period on the base... a very solemn reminder of the risks we faced every single minute of every single day.

I was in a state of suspended consequence, never knowing if, when, where, or how my heart would beat its last and final beat. I was not quite prepared for that mindset. But I knew I had to make sense of the environment.

Despite my mind's logic screaming the truth that "none of this" made any sense, I simply had to make the environment palatable. I needed to make peace with my "self"; I needed to quiet that part of me that was mentally calculating the huge increase in the risk and associated likelihood that I would die within the next ten, twenty, or thirty days.

On the other hand, I absolutely *needed* to believe I would **not** die. I wanted to escape every possible thought of death. For sanity's sake, war induced me to choose between fearing the possible... and living the probable.

Believe it or not, despite the increased risk of dying while in Iraq, my *chances for survival* were far greater. Moreover, as much as the risk of dying increases in a war zone, death actually stalks us every minute of every day.

THE MILITARY MANUAL
TO STOP SMOKING ASAP

Undeniably, death appears to shadow the elderly. But, in general, death has no favorite population. Though morbidity rates vary from country to country, death thrives among men, women, children, and among every race and nationality.

Accordingly, as you read this little book, you have the same invitation to the afterworld as the American Soldier deployed to a warzone.

As a smoker, you are an ideal candidate for death. In fact, every smoker is in a war with time. Seconds, minutes, days, and weeks are neither friend nor foe. As a smoker, however, time soon becomes your constant enemy.

As a smoker, it's just a matter of time before your quality of life begins to significantly deteriorate.

Sooner or later, even your denial will die, and you, too, will soon face the harsh reality that smoking cigarettes is a deadly act of denial.

As a smoker...

   Your denial has no set time of attack.

THE MILITARY MANUAL
TO STOP SMOKING ASAP

Sometimes the small smoke bombs explode into your lungs one at a time. During other self-inflicted attacks, the toxic smoke flows into your lungs, one after another for as long as an hour or so... often longer.

After the poisonous smoke is blasted into your lungs, there is a "blackout period" when your mind's rational thought process is shut down, feeding your denial as you reject the likelihood that doctors will someday notify your next-of-kin (as doctors have done with **all** the other smokers who have been killed by your enemy's slow-but-successful attacks).

No phone calls, e-mails, or other messages to you will be allowed once friends and family are notified of your smoking-related death.

Today, you are in a state of suspended consequence, not knowing if or when you will get cancer. Indeed, in your current state of denial, nothing can prepare you for such a cancerous existence. As you continue to smoke, your mind is trying to make sense of your self-created environment of destruction. Despite your mind's logic screaming the ugly truth that smoking dangerous toxins makes absolutely no sense, your super-strong denial is making your smoky environment palatable. In reality...

You are at war with your true self.

THE MILITARY MANUAL
TO STOP SMOKING ASAP

Every day... on a daily basis.. you make war and peace with your "self." You are conquering the part of you that is logically calculating the enormous increase in the likelihood that you will die within the next ten, twenty, or thirty years... from smoking-related illnesses.

Smokers *need* to believe they will not die. Smokers want to escape the thought of death. Quite literally, for sanity's sake, smoking causes you to choose between living a healthy life and living a life that will probably end with a cancerous disease. If you smoke, death stalks you wherever you roam. *Knock, knock...*

As you may already **know**, smoking your cigarettes has already significantly degraded the quality of your life. And, more importantly, as you continue to smoke, the quality of your life will get consistently worse.

Yes... if you smoke... **you** are in denial about the future quality of your life being affected by your actions of today. *"Reality" is the opposite of denial.* And, in reality, there is no rational reason for you to participate in such a death-loving behavior (smoking)... unless you are in a very dark death-spiral of denial.

Never underestimate the Power of Denial!

THE MILITARY MANUAL
TO STOP SMOKING ASAP

A classic study in denial is found in the story of passengers' actions aboard RMS Titanic, a huge luxury ship that sank in the cold waters of the North Atlantic Ocean in 1912.

The ship was considered unsinkable.

Unfortunately, on April 15, 1912, despite being warned that the ship was taking on excessive amounts of water, many of the passengers refused to accept the fact that the ship was sinking. Perhaps you have seen movies or heard the tales of passengers who refused to believe the ship was capable of being brought down by an iceberg.

Many of the passengers believed the Titanic was actually unsinkable. They were in denial.

If you were on a ship in the middle of the North Atlantic Ocean (a very cold ocean with big floating icebergs), would you simply wave good-bye and blow a kiss into the chilly night air as your loved ones departed on a lifeboat?

Would you hold fast to your faith in the unsinkable ship? Or would you slowly begin to accept reality? Because the passengers of the Titanic did not **accept** the reality of the situation, more than a thousand passengers did not adapt to the evolving situation.

THE MILITARY MANUAL
TO STOP SMOKING ASAP

They did not **accept** the fact that the ship was sinking. And since they did not adapt to the life-threatening conditions, many passengers failed to achieve a successful escape. In fact, one could say those passengers died of denial.

The same can be said about someone sitting in a smoke-filled room, refusing to accept the adage "where there's smoke, there's fire."

By accepting the possibility of a nearby fire, one can adapt to the dangerous situation and then seek an immediate exit. *Accepting* and *adapting* to the situation **creates** a higher probability of *achieving* survivability. Some people think "understanding" is more important than "acceptance." To them I ask:

> *"Do you* understand *how your television remote works? Do you* understand *the electronic interaction between the circuitry on the remote and the receiver on the television? Or, like most people, do you simply* 'accept' *that, if you push the 'on' button, the television will turn on?"*

We don't *understand* the electronic circuitry of the TV remote; we simply **accept** the technology and use it. The same is true with our acceptance & understanding of cigarettes.

THE MILITARY MANUAL TO STOP SMOKING ASAP

For too long, our society has accepted cigarettes, without fully understanding the facts related to the deaths caused by smoking.

This little book is not about today's society.

This little book is about getting **you** to accept this fact: smoking causes lung cancer and heart disease. By **accepting** this fact, and then **adapting** to a smoking-cessation plan based on these facts, you can **create** a clear path to **achieving** a healthier, smoke-free life.

Know this:

> *You are the **creator** of the next step. You are the **creator** of the rest of your life. If you keep smoking, you **create** death. If you stop smoking, you literally **create** a whole new life.*

As the receiver of the tremendous gift of life, you are responsible for protecting your great gift. Your fundamental mission is to **create** a style of life, a lifestyle, to protect your body, prepare your children, and prolong your time with your body and your children.

Smoking cigarettes destroys your body and shortens your time with people who love you. That's a fact. It's time to do the right thing.

It's time to quit smoking today!

THE MILITARY MANUAL
TO STOP SMOKING ASAP

Here is the Big Picture of this Little Book...

A. *Accept* a few facts.
  ▪ You **will** quit smoking.
  ▪ Keep smoking and you will die.
  ▪ People & products are against you.
  ▪ Smoking is not about nicotine.
  ▪ Smoking is based on specific desires.

B. *Adapt* your life to the above facts.
  ▪ Keep good habits, not the tobacco.
  ▪ Change your mind; educate it.

C. *Achieve* what you want.
  1. Choose your target; state your goal.
  2. Aim for the target.
  3. Focus on the target.
  4. Shoot/Find your way to the target.
  5. Assess distance/path to the target.
  6. Adjust your path to the target.
  7. Repeat step #5 and #6 until #8.
  8. Achieve your stated goal.
  9. Share your success story.
  10. Move on to your next goal!

The next twenty-five pages expand upon the Big Picture points above. As you read the next 25 pages, spend some time reminding yourself of this one great truth. Say it loudly:

~ What I *believe* is true (to me) ~

THE MILITARY MANUAL TO STOP SMOKING ASAP

Interestingly Enough

Of the three primary points on the previous page, the third item, *"Achieve what you want"* is actually the best place to start your efforts to quit smoking. Interestingly, when we see the word *achievement,* we usually think about the completion of a project.

Goal a*chievement,* however, is something we should envision first. And, as *you* embark on this smoking cessation program today, ask *your* **self** four simple questions:

So, what if it is true?
What can I do about it?
What will I do about it?
What AM I DOING about it?

To facilitate your transition from unhealthy smoker to healthy non-smoker, what are you doing this very moment to achieve your goal? Well, for starters, you are reading this book. Great! What's next? If this is step #1 (and it is), what happens when you finish reading this book? If you have about 20 minutes, the last 24 pages of this powerful little book can help you proudly say, *"I quit smoking!"*

If you smoke, you are already a statistic...

But being a statistic can be a good thing...

THE MILITARY MANUAL
TO STOP SMOKING ASAP

> ***20 minutes after you smoke your last cigarette, your body begins a series of changes that continue for years...***

- 20 minutes later, your heart rate drops.

- 12 hours later, carbon monoxide levels in your blood drops to normal.

- 2 weeks later, your heart-attack risk drops, and your lung function improves.

- 1 month later, expect your coughing and shortness of breath to decrease greatly.

- 1 year later, your added risk of coronary heart disease is half that of a smoker's.

- 5 years later, your stroke risk is reduced.

- 10 years later, the lung cancer death rate is about half that of a smoker's death rate.

- 15 years later, your risk of coronary heart disease is back to that of a nonsmoker's.

(Visit cdc.gov for additional facts to help you)

Has it been **20 minutes** since your last cigarette? If it has, you have already quit smoking. You are already a successful non-smoker. You can already say to yourself and others around you...

"I quit smoking!"

THE MILITARY MANUAL TO STOP SMOKING ASAP

Accept a Few Facts!

Remember: it's important to finish this entire book from beginning to end, straight through.

You can quit smoking today if you can consistently do three very specific things:

1. **Accept** a few facts.
2. **Adapt** your life to those facts.
3. **Achieve** what you want.

Accept a few facts: You *can* stop smoking, one way or another. Here's one way: Keep smoking and you will die. There... I said it. There. You read it. Read it again... aloud:

> ## "If I keep smoking, I <u>will</u> die."

Do you really want to die from smoking?

Over the years, I've heard many of the stupid, worn-out reasons for continuing to smoke. Some of the worst reasons include:

> "Not everyone who smokes will get cancer."
>
> "We must die from something.
> I might as well *choose* how I die."
>
> "I **like** to smoke; it relaxes me."

THE MILITARY MANUAL
TO STOP SMOKING ASAP

Accept this fact:

*Odds, **money**, & industry are against you.*

1. You will eventually quit smoking.
2. Keep smoking and you will die.
3. The odds are stacked against you... and so are people, products, and policies.

The tobacco industry has long been at the forefront of subliminal advertising. So, before you **think** about quitting the habit of smoking, you should **know** there is a constant barrage of cigarette advertising attacking your subconscious mind. Don't be alarmed about this fact; accept it and move on.

According to the *Center for Disease Control and Prevention* (CDC), the American tobacco industry has focused on women by producing brands with themes of social desirability and independence, which are conveyed by advertisements featuring slender, eye-catching, and (ironically) healthy models.

The CDC notes that marketing to Hispanics and Native Americans has included the creation of cigarette brands creatively named Rio, Dorado, and American Spirit.

To further facilitate subliminal acceptance of these products, the tobacco industry has sponsored various cultural events commemorating ethnic pride (rodeos, parades, festivals, etc.).

THE MILITARY MANUAL
TO STOP SMOKING ASAP

In districts with a significant population of minorities, the industry has used urban culture, language, and direct mail to promote menthol cigarettes. Tobacco-sponsored hip-hop bar nights (with samples of menthol cigarettes) have also been used for this effort.

All children continue to be at risk. In 2006, the three most heavily advertised brands (Marlboro, Newport, and Camel) were the favored brand name of cigarettes smoked by high-school and middle-school teen smokers.

That same year, cigarette companies spent $12.4 billion on advertising and promotional expenses in the United States (double the amount spent in 1997). To put these figures in perspective, the CDC estimates cigarette companies spent about **$34 million per day** on U.S. marketing efforts. That's at least $275 for each U.S. smoker over 18 years old!

With that much money thrown into the marketing equation, the odds are stacked against you... and so are people, products, and policies. Friends and family members have seen you "quit before," and they may not be your best supporters. Additionally, the policies of many medical insurance plans pay for smoking cessation *drugs*, but don't really provide a *plan* to successfully stop smoking.

THE MILITARY MANUAL
TO STOP SMOKING ASAP

Today, those other people, products, and policies don't matter. Today, **you** are the only thing that matters. You are the power to quit.

Notice the wording of the previous sentence:

~ You *are* the power to stop smoking! ~

The sentence above does not say, "You *have* the power to stop smoking." In reality, you *are* the power; this is a fact. Accept it and move on. You don't need anything or anybody else to help you quit. You have everything you need right here: YOU.

You are at war with your true self.

Today is the day to make peace with your self. Ask yourself: *if I could have only **one** or the other, which would I rather have: all the money in the world or all the time in the world?*

In reality, we can't have either one. However, here's a related question: *if I could have only **one** or the other, which one would I rather have: $86,400 a day or 86,400 seconds a day?*

As the creator of the next second, minute, hour, and day of your life, you are the one who decides what to do with your money and your time. You are already wealthy because every day is full of 86,400 seconds.

The question is,

"What will you do with your time?"

THE MILITARY MANUAL
TO STOP SMOKING ASAP

Accept a Few Facts:

1. You *can* quit smoking.
2. Keep smoking and you will die.
3. The odds are stacked against you.
4. Desire to smoke is not about nicotine.

According to Wikipedia.com:

> *Addiction has been defined with regard solely to psychoactive substances (alcohol, tobacco and other drugs) which cross the blood-brain barrier once ingested, temporarily altering the chemical environment of the brain.*

For me, smoking is NOT an addiction.
I had to stop calling it an "addiction."

Your desire to smoke is not about smoking. Your desire to smoke is just that: a desire.

Owning your choice to smoke is important. When people say they are addicted, they are surrendering to a totally integrated life with their choice of habit. Choose reality; reject denial, and call it what it is: ***smoking is a choice.*** Calling it something else takes power from you and gives it to the "addiction."

Though not a medical doctor, here's the view from John Clark III, a former Commander in the United States Navy who enlisted in the Navy and smoked cigarettes for well over 15 years:

THE MILITARY MANUAL
TO STOP SMOKING ASAP

Desire to smoke might not be about nicotine.

Your desire may be just that: a desire; a want.

Currently, you probably *want* to smoke.

Remove the desire. You *will* stop smoking.

It's just that simple.

Patches, people, products, and policies are crutches that will soon surrender to **your** desire to smoke one cigarette... and then another, and then another, etc.

Patches, gum, or lozenges will not solve the problem of your desire. Accept a few facts:

1. You *can* quit smoking.
2. Keep smoking and you will die.
3. People, products, policies are against you.
4. Your desire to smoke isn't about nicotine.
5. Your desire to smoke is likely based on three basic concepts:
   a. **Physical**
   b. **Physiological**
   c. **Mental**

Let's address the *physical* aspects of smoking.

A textbook definition of the word *physical* is:

> *"Having substance or material existence; perceptible to the senses."*

THE MILITARY MANUAL
TO STOP SMOKING ASAP

Thus, the physical aspects of smoking include the bodily preparations.

Some examples include walking to the designated smoke area; reaching for the pack of cigarettes; pulling out the cigarette; igniting the tobacco; inhaling the deadly smoke; exhaling the less-deadly smoke; and, in general, "*all the* physical *things associated with smoking.*"

As you probably already know, the physical mechanics of doing anything can become habitual if you do it long enough.

For example, if you start watching the morning news at 6am every day for a year, you will develop a strong physical tendency to awake just before 6am everyday... physically adapted to watching the 6am news.

The physiological aspects, on the other hand, are related to the mechanical, physical, and biochemical processes of humans. Thus, physiology is the "software" behind the physical (hardware) activity of bodily movement.

The **physiological** aspects of smoking can only be achieved after prolonged physical attraction to the process of smoking. Likewise, once the physical crosses into the physiological, your capability to quit smoking requires more than a passing effort.

THE MILITARY MANUAL
TO STOP SMOKING ASAP

Your capability to quit smoking requires a proactive process that actively does two things: 1) smacks you out of denial; and 2) directly addresses the physical, physiological, and mental threats to your success.

First, let's address the denial...

With regard to psychological discussions, *denial* is a subconscious defense mechanism characterized by refusal to acknowledge painful realities, thoughts, or feelings.

In other words, when we are in denial about something, we are actually in an alternate reality; **we are actively choosing to live a lie.**

Interestingly enough, if I were to ask you, *"What are YOU in denial about?"* What do you think you would you say?

In reality, YOU are not qualified to answer that question. By definition, "denial" is a subconscious (**mental**) thought process. It is a thought-based decision to reject certain facts.

Denial is a refusal to see or accept reality.

So... today, with this book, YOU begin the powerfully proactive process to address your denial. YOU are in control of when YOU stop smoking. Keep smoking, and YOU will die.

Let's review a few facts and simple questions.

THE MILITARY MANUAL TO STOP SMOKING ASAP

You can quit smoking. Keep smoking and you will die. People and products are against you. Your desire to smoke is based on three specific characteristics: physical, physiological, and mental. These are the facts. Accept them and move on.

Based on the facts above, let's review four simple questions and form our simple plan:

So, what if the facts above are true?

> **What can YOU do about it?**
>
> **What will YOU do about it?**

What are **YOU** *doing about it?*

If you can *accept* the **bold** facts above, you can *adapt* to those facts. And if you can adapt to those facts, you can actually begin the process to move beyond denial. As you move beyond denial, you can make peace with your self; no more war!

Can you see the beginning of your plan? There's more to follow. But, first: Accept the facts. Adapt accordingly. And then you can truly *achieve* a smoke-free life! Has it been 20 minutes yet? Awesome!

Accept, adapt, say...

"I quit smoking!"

THE MILITARY MANUAL
TO STOP SMOKING ASAP

Adapt Accordingly

Your **threats** to successfully quit smoking must be addressed. What does this mean?

This simply means YOU should not ignore those things that directly affect and undermine YOUR ability to quit smoking. Face these challenges! HOW will YOU do this?

There is a really good way to do this... Take those threats and turn them into assets (or support mechanisms).

For example, as a smoker, you are probably...

1. *Physically* accustomed to taking a (smoke) break every hour or so;

2. *Physically* accustomed to doing things integrated with your hands and mouth;

3. *Physically* accustomed to inhaling deeply, and exhaling methodically;

4. *Physically* accustomed to certain small rituals associated with prepping for your (smoke) break.

Let's address the physical threats to success.

THE MILITARY MANUAL TO STOP SMOKING ASAP

As YOU begin a smoke-free life, those same *physical* tendencies will not just *go away*. Those same physical tendencies will tend to work against your newfound desire to stop smoking. So instead of ignoring the threats, let's face those tendencies and use them as **assets** to actually help you quit smoking.

1. **Take your breaks.** Since you are *physically* accustomed to taking a (smoke) break every hour, keep the habit of taking breaks. However, instead of going to the smoking area, go in another direction, literally. Where you go is unimportant. Keeping the break habit *is* important.

   As a smoker, you have conditioned your body to consistently expect a break every hour (or whatever your smoking frequency was). Don't disappoint your self. Keep the good (break) habit; stop the bad (smoking) habit. *You can do this!*

2. **Go through the motions.** Since you are physically accustomed to doing things with your hands and mouth, continue this habit, but do it with something as harmless as air. Instead of a cigarette, cut up and *inhale through a straw*.

   Let's call these straws "IQSTix"... IQ sticks (because you are too smart to keep smoking). Also, IQST stands for...

   "I quit smoking today!"

THE MILITARY MANUAL TO STOP SMOKING ASAP

3. **"Smoke" clean air.** Since you are physically accustomed to inhaling deeply and exhaling methodically, don't disappoint your self. Take your breaks; inhale all that great fresh air through your fake cigarette. Then, exhale methodically, just like you did when you *were* a smoker. Imagine your lungs pinking up as you breathe in all that pure healthy air.

4. **Keep your rituals.** Since you are physically accustomed to certain small rituals connected with prepping for your (smoke) break, do the same thing with your IQSTix. Keep your IQSTix in a valued place. Carefully remove one IQSTix at a time. Don't just *give* your IQSTix away. And, if you so desire, feel free to use more than one IQSTix during your break. *This may sound hokey; but it really works!*

Consistently doing those four basic steps will help you adapt to these five basic facts:

1. You will stop smoking one way or another
2. Here's one way: smoke and you will die
3. The odds are stacked against you
4. Desire to smoke is not about nicotine
5. Your desire to smoke is based on three concepts: *physical habits, physiological connections, and mental acceptance.*

THE MILITARY MANUAL
TO STOP SMOKING ASAP

Remember...

1. **Take your breaks.**
2. **Go through the motions.**
3. **"Smoke" clean air.**
4. **Keep your rituals.**

As you start this awesome, life-saving program, focus on your target: *I have stopped smoking.* And, just like a bullet leaving the muzzle of a gun, you might miss the mark.

If this happens, simply adjust your aim and fire again. In other words, don't give up; align your aim; focus, and fire again.

Once you set and see your target goal, you can clearly see how close (or far) you are to hitting your mark. And when it comes to goal setting, smoking cessation, and hitting targets, *you will inevitably* hit the mark when you follow ten basic steps of goal achievement:

1. **Choose your target; state your goal!**
2. **Aim for the target.**
3. **Focus on the target!**
4. **Shoot/Find your way to the target.**
5. **Assess distance/path to the target.**
6. **Adjust your path to the target.**
7. **Repeat step #5 & #6 until you hit #8.**
8. **Achieve your stated goal!**
9. **Share your success story.**
10. **Move on to another goal.**

THE MILITARY MANUAL TO STOP SMOKING ASAP

Achieve Your Desired Results

Now that we have addressed the physical aspects of your desire to smoke, let's focus on the **physiological** and mental aspects.

Know this: The **physiological** part of you is actually the integration and coordination of the physical and mental aspects of you. In other words, the **physiological** part of you is where your physical and mental selves meet. It's where the brain meets the mind.

The **physiological** part of you is where your physical and mental selves argue. Fortunately for you, the **physiological** part of you is where your "physical and mental selves" also come into some form of agreement. So...

To successfully change from smoker to non-smoker, you must **CREATE AGREEMENT** between your mental and physical selves. To **create** agreement between your mental and physical selves, simply change your mind, and your body will follow. How? Simply accept the straight-forward facts about smoking. Think about this (*create* this thought): by accepting and adapting to facts, you **create** a clear, reality-based path to achievement. You can actually say...

"I Quit Smoking!"

THE MILITARY MANUAL
TO STOP SMOKING ASAP

As a smoker, your <u>mental</u> self (your mind) has been dominated by denial. In turn, your mind allows you to smoke toxin-filled cigarettes. However, as you move through this powerful little book, you are realizing the power you have over your denial. As you go forward, this powerful little book will show you how to become more powerful over your denial. Do you really want to quit smoking? All you have to do is change your mind.

Change your mind about smoking.

Have you ever decided to go see a particular movie and then, upon arriving at the theater, decided to see another (different) movie?

You simply changed your mind.

Have you ever decided to eat at the place that sells tacos, and then suddenly decided to eat at the place that sells burgers?

You simply changed your mind.

To truly quit smoking, all you have to do is change your mind. Remember: YOU are in control of what YOU do to YOUR body. Do not try to avoid this awesome responsibility. YOU are reading this book. Thus, YOU are able to respond to the recommended plans within this book. Yes, YOU are able to respond to this book. You are response-*able*.

Respond!

THE MILITARY MANUAL TO STOP SMOKING ASAP

You can change your mind about whether or not smoking is an okay thing to do. Deep down inside, you *know* it's not okay to smoke.

Today, with this book, YOU begin the proactive process to address your denial. YOU are in control of when YOU stop smoking. Keep smoking and YOU will die.

Thus far, we have addressed YOUR powerfully proactive process to actively 1) smack you out of denial; and 2) directly address the threats to your success.

We took those threats and discovered how to turn them into assets (doing similar physical activities while replacing cigarettes with items to support your goal to stop smoking).

Getting over the physical habit of smoking seems especially challenging for some people. And getting over the mental habit seems harder for others. So... what do I mean when I say, *"Simply change your mind"*?

After all, quitting smoking is nothing like going to the movies! And, changing the feature attraction is not at all related to killing YOUR self slowly... *or is it?* Change your mind; see a different movie. Change your mind; live a longer life. The similarities are real.

In reality, your life is a series of movies.

THE MILITARY MANUAL
TO STOP SMOKING ASAP

You are the star. You are the director!

Moreover, your life is a series of experiments. There is almost nothing permanent about YOU! Your skin, your eyes, your mind, and your mouth... they all change over time.

And, yes... you are not a permanent smoker! You can change from a smoker to a non-smoker. I did it, and so did millions of other people. But how can this change occur?

Who makes the changes occur in YOUR life?

YOU make the changes happen!
YOU either cause or allow things to occur.

What does this mean?

This simply means YOU are the creator of your life. This simply means YOU must not ignore those things that directly affect and undermine YOUR ability to quit smoking.

How can YOU conquer denial?

There is only one good way to do this: take the mental threat of denial totally out of your thinking process. Smack yourself into reality.

THE MILITARY MANUAL
TO STOP SMOKING ASAP

To achieve a smoke-free life, the best way to address the mental challenge of denial is to confront it "head-on." How can you do this?

E D U C A T I O N !

The most effective way to change your mind is to educate your self. Read, research, and renegotiate the agreements between your mind and your heart. Read, research, and replace your current thoughts and feelings about cigarettes. Read, research, and reveal to your self the absolutely horrific damage you are doing to your body every time you suck on one of those disgusting sticks of cancer-causing, creators of death and sorrow.

Would you buy a car without researching and reviewing the relevant safety information? Would you buy a house without knowing how much the commitment could cost you? Most people will keep a car for 3-5 years. Many homeowners will keep their house for 10-20 years. How long will you keep your body?

Why would you purposely suck on known carcinogens without researching the life-threatening effects they can have on your body? If you really want to quit smoking, change your mind.

Eliminate your denial!

THE MILITARY MANUAL TO STOP SMOKING ASAP

Let's not get confused by the facts here.

Indeed, you can educate your true self on almost anything. And by searching the vast Internet and your local library, you can gain fantastic knowledge about the dangers of smoking.

However, there is a significant difference between *knowledge* and *wisdom*.

Knowledge is made of mere facts, figures, and forgetful information. *Wisdom*, on the other hand, is the actual application of knowledge. Accordingly, you can be the smartest person on earth (in terms of how much knowledge you have). But, if you don't use that knowledge, you are the "most unwise" person in the world! Knowledge is transformed into wisdom only when you ***use*** *the knowledge.*

YOU are transformed from a knowledgeable smoker into a wise non-smoker only when you use your knowledge about the dangers of smoking, and say *"I quit smoking!"*

Yes... you can quit smoking today if you do three specific things:

1. *Accept* **a few facts**
2. *Adapt* **your life to those facts**
3. *Achieve* **a non-smoking life**

The next 3 pages are now **<u>YOUR</u>** reality...

THE MILITARY MANUAL TO STOP SMOKING ASAP

I have accepted these facts:

1. I **will** quit smoking, one way or another.
2. Here's one way: keep smoking; I will die.
3. The odds are stacked against me...
4. My desire to smoke is not about nicotine.
5. My desire to smoke is based on 3 things:
    a. Physical; Physiological; Mental

I have adapted to the following actions:

1. **Take my breaks.** I am physically accustomed to taking an occasional break. I will keep this healthy hourly habit.

   However, instead of walking to my designated smoke area, I will go in the opposite direction. I will choose a new path. Keeping this hourly habit is important. My body wants to take an occasional break. I won't disappoint myself. I will keep the good habit and take an occasional break. I have stopped the bad habit. *"I quit smoking!"*

2. **Go through the motions.** I am physically accustomed to doing things associated with my hands and my mouth. Instead of using cigarettes, I will use IQSTix. As I consistently adapt my physical motions, I will continuously, consciously say to my self, *"I quit smoking!"*

THE MILITARY MANUAL TO STOP SMOKING ASAP

3. **"Smoke" clean air.** I am physically accustomed to inhaling deeply, and then exhaling methodically. I won't disappoint my self. I will take my breaks. As I inhale and exhale, I will imagine my lungs pinking up as I breathe in smoke-free air.

4. **Keep my rituals.** Since I am physically accustomed to certain small rituals associated with prepping for my breaks, I will do the same thing with my IQSTix. Today, I gladly say to my new non-smoking self, *"I quit smoking!"*

5. **Change my mind.** I am educating myself about the damage smoking does to my body. I will focus on finding information. I will seek information as if my life depends on it. Why? Because my life depends on my ability to change my mind. And the best way to change my mind is to educate myself. My mind *has* changed.

   - *To educate myself, change my mind, and remind myself of the deadly details about smoking, I will keep factual, quick-reference cards with me. (visit www.johnclarkiii.com/ASAP)*

   - *When I believe or think I want a cigarette, I will make the choice to take my break, walk my path, and accept my reality that I choose not to smoke...*

   - *I choose to live a long, healthy life.*

THE MILITARY MANUAL TO STOP SMOKING ASAP

Your Final Statement. Say It...

In the real world of here and now, there is no such thing as yesterday or. Yesterday does not actually exist, and my tomorrow may never arrive. There is only right here, right now.

And then there **is** the miracle that **is** me.

I **am** a miraculous gift of life. My life is not made up of cool characters and slick slogans as seen in cigarette advertisements. My life **is** made of breaths and lungs; hearts and beats; thoughts and actions; and hugs & kisses. My one-and-only life **is** made of this great day.

Today **is** the day I begin my new life that honors all 86,400 seconds of my day by breathing clean air, nursing my only beating heart, and acting on my fact-based thoughts.

In the final analysis, my loved ones have no control over my lungs, my heart, or my brain. Those special organs only play music for me.

Hugs and kisses, however, are given to me because my loved ones want me here for a very long time. But if cancer takes my life, my loved ones will be left with nothing but smoke-filled memories. So... as I finish this great little book, I have made the life-saving choice to tell them...

"I quit smoking!"

THE MILITARY MANUAL TO STOP SMOKING ASAP

About The Author

Other books by John H. Clark III:

The Ideal:
Your Guide to An Ideal Life

Getting Out:
Expert Advice for
Today's Teens

God's Heartbeat:
A Powerful Premise
for Leading a
Christian
Life

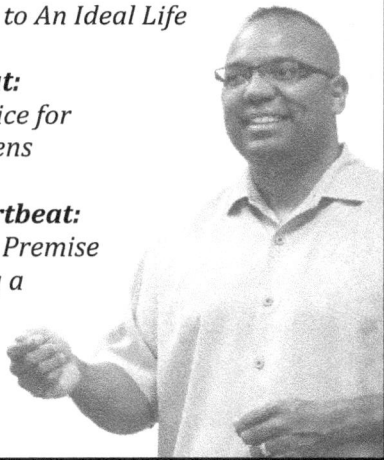

Dedicated to leveraging today's successes into investments for future leaders of our nation, John H. Clark III is founder of The PIE Group, a consulting firm focused on implementing successful change-management strategies.

www.johnclarkiii.com

www.ingramcontent.com/pod-product-compliance
Lightning Source LLC
Chambersburg PA
CBHW021338290326
41933CB00038B/973